Flexibility and Balance for Seniors

Unlock easy, holistic methods to prevent falls, enhance flexibility, restore mobility, and preserve your independence

Paul Fyneface

Disclaimer

This book, "Flexibility and Balance for Seniors," contains material that is solely meant to be used for informative and instructional reasons. The author and publisher make every effort to guarantee the truth and completeness of the material offered, but they do not accept liability for any errors, inaccuracies, or omissions. It is recommended that readers get advice from licensed healthcare providers before implementing any dietary, lifestyle, or exercise modifications based on the information presented here.

The information contained in this book is not meant to replace expert medical advice, diagnosis, or care. Before starting a new fitness, program or making big dietary or lifestyle changes, it is imperative to speak with your doctor or other certified healthcare professional.

To suit your unique fitness level, flexibility, and any potential physical restrictions or injuries, it is crucial to pay attention to your body and adjust workouts as necessary. Any pain, discomfort, or dizziness should be promptly stopped when exercising.

This book's nutritional data and dietary suggestions are only suggestions; they might not be appropriate for all readers. Depending on things like age, gender, degree of exercise, and medical history, each person may have different dietary demands. To create a customized nutrition plan that meets your unique requirements and objectives, it is advised that you speak with a licensed dietitian or nutritionist.

To reduce the chance of injury, exercise must be done in a secure setting with the right tools, using perfect form and technique. Ask a certified fitness expert or healthcare practitioner for advice if you are unclear about how to carry out a certain workout properly. Any liabilities or damages resulting from the use of the information included in this book are disclaimed by the author and publisher. Readers take all responsibility for their choices and behaviors about their health and welfare.

In conclusion, the goal of "Flexibility and Balance for Seniors" is to provide readers with the tools they need to take charge of their health and wellbeing by offering doable tactics and methods for boosting flexibility, balancing out, and encouraging general wellbeing. To protect your safety and wellbeing, you must, nonetheless, approach the information cautiously and get expert advice when necessary.

Table of Contents

Introduction

Introducing "Flexibility and Balance for Seniors," an all-inclusive manual for enhancing mobility, steadiness, and general health as we age gracefully. We go on an exploration of the significance of balance and flexibility for seniors in this book, along with useful tips and workouts to help you preserve and improve these vital components of physical well-being.

Maintaining balance and flexibility becomes more and more important as we traverse the golden years for our quality of life. Maintaining independence and vitality, avoiding falls and accidents, and carrying out everyday tasks all depend on these two aspects of physical fitness. On the other hand, a lot of seniors struggle with impaired balance and flexibility, which can cause mobility restrictions, low self-esteem, and an increased chance of falling.

You can maximize your flexibility and balance by following the instructions in this book, so don't worry. The knowledge and activities offered here are meant to empower you on your path to greater health and vitality, regardless of your age and ability to move about. Perhaps you are a caregiver trying to support the health of a loved one.

First, we will explore the principles of flexibility and balance in the upcoming chapters. We will go into the definitions of these phrases, their significance, and their effects on our day-to-day existence as elderly people. A foundation for the exercises and tactics we will talk about later is understanding the significance of flexibility and balance.

We'll then go into useful methods for enhancing flexibility. You'll learn several techniques to improve your range of motion and lessen stiffness and discomfort, from stretching exercises that target certain muscle areas to customized flexibility training regimens. You'll discover how to safely and successfully include flexibility exercises into your everyday routine with the aid of clear instructions and practical advice.

After that, we'll focus on training for balance. You'll discover how important balance is for keeping one's equilibrium and avoiding falls, especially as one becomes older. You will gain strength, coordination, and proprioception via a variety of balancing exercises and training regimens, which will enable you to walk confidently and steadily on your feet.

However, that's not all. The synergistic link between flexibility and balance is explored in this book, which goes beyond individual exercises. Learn how these two aspects of physical fitness complement each other to enhance overall quality of life and facilitate functional movement. You may get a higher degree of mobility, stability, and energy by including flexibility and balance exercises in your regular regimen.

The Importance of Flexibility and Balance in Aging

For general health and wellbeing, it becomes more and more crucial as we age to maintain flexibility and balance. Maintaining stability and control over our body's position is known as balance, whereas the capacity of our muscles and joints to move freely over their whole range of motion is referred to as flexibility. We'll discuss the importance of flexibility and balance in healthy aging in this part, as well as how they support independence, reduce the risk of falls, and improve quality of life in general.

Maintaining Independence:

As we go about our daily lives, we have to be able to bend over to tie our shoes, reach up high on shelves for items, and get in and out of seats, among other chores that need flexibility and balance. The ability to preserve independence and ease of performance in these tasks as we age is facilitated by the preservation of muscle and joint flexibility. The chance of mishaps and injuries is also decreased when we have good balance, which enables us to move through our surroundings with assurance and safety.

Preventing Falls:

Seniors are particularly concerned about fall risk since it can result in catastrophic injuries and consequences. Fall risk is greatly increased by poor flexibility and balance because the restricted range of motion and inflexible muscles can make it difficult to move around and coordinate. Seniors can lower their chance of falling and preserve their safety and well-being as they age by increasing their flexibility and balance via specific exercises and training.

Enhancing Mobility:

To keep the joints moving as freely and as comfortably as possible, flexibility and balance are crucial. We tend to have stiffer, more uncomfortable muscles as we age because they are less flexible and tighter. Further affecting our capacity to move confidently and effectively as we age are changes in proprioception and balance. Our everyday routines can benefit from regular flexibility and balancing exercises because they can help us move more freely and pleasantly as we age by reducing muscle tension, improving joint mobility, and enhancing overall mobility.

Supporting Joint Health:

Frequent stretches for flexibility aid in maintaining the range of motion and lubrication of the joints. This is especially crucial for elderly people since aging-related changes in the joints, such as a decline in cartilage and the formation of synovial fluid, can cause stiffness and decreased mobility. Seniors may maintain joint health and lower their chance of developing diseases like osteoarthritis and arthritis by performing focused stretching and mobility exercises to keep their joints supple and flexible.

Improving Posture and Alignment:

Maintaining proper posture and alignment is critical for general health and function, and these can only be achieved via flexibility and balance. Adequate posture can exacerbate musculoskeletal disorders such as back discomfort and muscular imbalances, whereas proper posture helps maintain an appropriate weight distribution and lessens the load on the joints and spine. Seniors can attain improved posture and alignment and lower their risk of discomfort and injury by strengthening their proprioception, balance, and flexibility in their tight muscles.

Flexibility and balance are crucial elements of good aging, promoting independence, mobility, and general well-being. We will discuss these issues throughout this trip as we address typical obstacles experienced by seniors. Seniors may lower their risk of falling, increase their mobility, and preserve their quality of life as they age by implementing specific exercises and training programs that promote flexibility and balance. Purchasing "Flexibility and Balance for Seniors" entitles investors to a thorough manual on long-term health and vitality, enabling them to age more gracefully and have better lives throughout their golden years.

Chapter One
Understanding Flexibility

Our capacity to move freely and carry out everyday tasks with ease is greatly influenced by flexibility, which is a basic requirement of physical fitness. We get into the details of flexibility in this chapter, explaining what it means, why it matters, and how it affects our general health and wellbeing. We may improve our quality of life and increase our range of motion by developing a greater grasp of flexibility.

What is Flexibility?

The term "flexibility" describes our musculoskeletal system's capacity to move freely across its whole range of motion without experiencing pain or limitation. It includes both static flexibility, which is maintaining a stretch in a fixed posture, and dynamic flexibility, which is carefully extending and contracting the joints to their maximum range of motion. Numerous factors, such as age, gender, physical activity level, heredity, and lifestyle choices, all have an impact on flexibility.

The Benefits of Flexibility

An important factor in preserving general health and wellbeing in the context of exercise is flexibility, which is sometimes disregarded. Flexibility has several advantages that go well beyond physical mobility, such as the ability to do amazing yoga postures or even just touch your toes. We will examine the many benefits of flexibility in this part, providing insight into the reasons that regular exercise programs must include flexibility training.

Increased Range of Motion:

The improvement of our range of motion is one of the main advantages of flexibility. Our ability to do daily tasks more effortlessly and effectively is enhanced when our muscles and joints are flexible since they can move through their whole range of motion more readily. Greater flexibility makes it possible for us to move more freely and easily in our daily lives, whether it is reaching for items on high shelves, bending down to tie our shoes, or engaging in recreational activities.

Reduced Risk of Injury:

The capacity of our bodies to absorb shock and adjust to abrupt movements is enhanced by flexibility, which is why it is so important in preventing injuries. Particularly during physical exercise or sports, tight muscles and limited range of motion can raise the risk of sprains, strains, and other musculoskeletal problems. Regular stretching and mobility exercises help us maintain optimal flexibility, which lowers the risk of injury and lessens the effects of wear and strain on our joints and soft tissues.

Improved Posture and Alignment:

Flexibility also contributes to better posture and alignment, which are essential for overall musculoskeletal health. Poor posture, characterized by rounded shoulders, forward head posture, and an arched lower back, can lead to muscle imbalances, spinal misalignment, and chronic pain. By improving flexibility in tight muscles and strengthening weak muscles, we can correct postural deviations, alleviate discomfort, and promote better spinal alignment, leading to improved posture and overall body mechanics.

Enhanced Athletic Performance:

To maximize performance and reach their full athletic potential, athletes and fitness fanatics must be flexible. Increased power and force production, better form and technique maintenance during practice and competition are all made possible by increased flexibility in athletes. In addition, flexibility training helps lessen pain in the muscles, minimize overuse injuries, and speed up the recovery process after workouts—all of which enable athletes to push themselves harder and reach their maximum potential.

Stress Relief and Relaxation:

Deep breathing, mindfulness, and body awareness are encouraged by flexibility activities like yoga and light stretching, which help people unwind and relieve tension. To alleviate stress, worry, and mental exhaustion, stretching helps to release tension from the muscles and soothe the neurological system. We may promote relaxation and general well-being by including flexibility exercises in our daily routine, which can offer a much-needed break from the stresses of life.

Thus, there are several advantages that flexibility provides for our mental, emotional, and physical well-being. Athletic performance, stress alleviation, better posture, and a broader range of motion are just a few benefits. We may improve our general quality of life and take advantage of all the benefits that flexibility has to offer by making flexibility a priority and including frequent stretching and mobility exercises in our daily routine.

Common Age-Related Flexibility Issues

Several physiological changes that occur to our bodies as we age may have an impact on our range of motion. To preserve general health and well-being as we traverse the aging process, it is essential to comprehend these age-related flexibility difficulties. This section will look at some of the most typical age-related flexibility problems and offer solutions and mitigation techniques for these difficulties.

Decreased Muscle Elasticity:

A decline in muscular suppleness is one of the main problems with age-related flexibility. Our muscles often lose some of their pliability and resistance to stretching as we age. It may become harder to carry out daily tasks and preserve ideal mobility as a result of this elasticity loss, which can also cause stiffness, tightness, and a decreased range of motion. Additionally, especially during physical activity or exercise, muscle stiffness can raise the risk of strains, sprains, and other injuries.

Stiffening of Connective Tissues:

Aging also affects the flexibility of our connective tissues, which include ligaments and tendons, in addition to changes in muscle elasticity. With aging, these tissues typically lose some of their flexibility and become more susceptible to adhesions and stiffness. Increased stiffness, pain, and difficulty moving can result from this connective tissue stiffening, which can also limit joint mobility and range of motion.

Loss of Muscle Mass:

Sarcopenia, or the decrease of muscular mass, is another age-related problem with flexibility. Our bodies naturally change as we age, resulting in a loss of muscular mass and strength among other things. In addition to raising the risk of falls and fractures, this loss of muscle mass can lead to decreased flexibility and movement. Reduced muscle mass can also result in imbalances in the muscles and changes in the way that the body moves, which can impair flexibility and the quality of movements in general.

Joint Stiffness and Degeneration:

The aging process can also affect flexibility and mobility due to joint changes including osteoarthritis and cartilage degradation. Specifically, osteoarthritis is a prevalent ailment that impairs joints, resulting in discomfort, rigidity, and diminished mobility. Every joint loses some of its flexibility and becomes more prone to pain and stiffness as the cartilage in the joint ages. It may be extremely difficult to carry out daily tasks and have an active lifestyle as a result, seriously reducing mobility and quality of life.

Sedentary Lifestyle:

Ultimately, one of the main causes of age-related flexibility problems is a sedentary lifestyle. Maintaining flexibility, strength, and mobility as we age requires us to be physically active and exercise regularly. Nonetheless, a lot of seniors could become less active over time as a result of things like retirement, long-term medical ailments, or mobility problems. Age-related flexibility problems can be made worse by a lack of regular physical exercise, which can result in additional loss of flexibility, muscular weakness, and reduced mobility.

Therefore, preserving general mobility and well-being as well as encouraging healthy aging require an awareness of the prevalent age-related flexibility difficulties. Seniors can increase flexibility, lessen stiffness and discomfort, and improve their general quality of life by treating these problems with focused flexibility exercises, strength training, and regular physical activity.

Flexibility Assessments and Tests

Before setting out on a quest to increase flexibility, it's critical to assess our existing situation and pinpoint any potential improvement areas. Tests and examinations of flexibility offer important insights into our range of motion, emphasizing our strong points and potential problem areas. This section will discuss popular tests and evaluations for flexibility that are used to gauge a person's level of flexibility and provide direction for programs that teach it.

Sit-and-Reach Test:

Flexibility of the lower back and hamstrings may be evaluated with ease using the sit-and-reach test. Seated on the floor, with your feet flat against a box or wall, execute this test by extending your legs straight in front of you. Without bending your knees, slowly extend both hands forward and slide them as far down the floor as you can. Find out how flexible you are by measuring the distance you've achieved and comparing it to standard charts.

Shoulder Flexibility Test:

Shoulder and upper back range of motion is evaluated with the shoulder flexibility test. Standing tall and extending your arms shoulder-height to the sides is how you should conduct this exam. Gently fold your arms in front of your body, ensuring that they are crossed at the wrist. To gauge your shoulder's flexibility, measure the space between your fingertips and compare it to established charts.

Hip Flexibility Test:

The hip flexor and joint range of motion are assessed using the hip flexibility test. Lay flat on your back with one leg stretched straight and the other bent at the knee, and place your foot flat on the ground to complete this test. Lift your bent knee slowly toward your chest while maintaining a level floor with your other leg. Hip flexibility may be evaluated by measuring the angle that forms between the outstretched leg and the floor.

Trunk Rotation Test:

Spine and trunk range of motion is measured via the trunk rotation exam. Place your legs out in front of you straight while sitting on the floor to complete this exam. Lay one foot flat on the ground outside the knee of the other person and cross it over the other. Reach back with the opposing arm by swiveling your body to the bent knee. To determine the trunk's flexibility, measure the degree of rotation and compare it to official charts.

Flexibility Training Programs:

People can customize their flexibility training programs to target certain areas of imbalance and weakness based on the findings of flexibility tests and evaluations. A range of stretching exercises that target various muscle groups and joints are commonly included in flexibility training regimens. Static and dynamic stretches as well as proprioceptive neuromuscular facilitation (PNF) techniques are a few examples of these exercises that may be done regularly to progressively increase flexibility.

Tests and evaluations of flexibility are important resources for determining one's degree of flexibility and directing training initiatives. To address particular requirements and increase the range of motion generally, people can create customized flexibility training regimens by recognizing their areas of imbalance and deficiency.

Chapter Two
Improving Flexibility

In this chapter, we go more deeply into the methods and approaches for enhancing flexibility, which is essential for preserving mobility and general health, particularly as we age. We examine how to safely and progressively enhance flexibility, increasing more range of movement and lowering the chance of injury, with an emphasis on mild, efficient exercises designed specifically for seniors. You may realize your ability to move confidently and with ease by implementing these flexibility-enhancing exercises into your daily routine.

Stretching Techniques for Seniors

Being flexible is more and more crucial as we get older for retaining mobility, lowering the chance of injury, and improving our general quality of life. You may improve your range of motion, reduce stiffness, and encourage improved alignment and posture by adding mild stretching exercises to your regimen. Let's examine each of these stretching methods in more depth.

Static Stretching:

Maintaining a stretch for a certain amount of time allows the muscles and connective tissues to progressively lengthen.

This technique is known as static stretching. Seniors may safely and effectively increase their flexibility with this kind of stretching since it doesn't place undue strain on their joints. To optimize results and reduce discomfort, we'll go over how to do static stretches for different muscle groups, with special emphasis on alignment and good technique.

Dynamic Stretching:

With dynamic stretching, the body is moved gently and repeatedly through a range of motion in a controlled manner. Dynamic stretching, as opposed to static stretching, aids in boosting blood flow, warming up the muscles, and getting the body ready for exercise. We'll look at dynamic stretching exercises that are appropriate for seniors, emphasizing fluid motions that increase range of motion and flexibility without putting the body under stress or risk of harm.

Proprioceptive Neuromuscular Facilitation (PNF) Stretching:

PNF stretching is a more complex stretching method that increases flexibility by having the muscles alternate between contracted and relaxed. While some seniors may not benefit from PNF stretching, there are modified versions of these techniques that can help with range of motion and flexibility. We'll go over partner assistance in stretches, the use of props for stability and support, and safe techniques for executing mild PNF stretching exercises.

Yoga-Based Stretching:

Stretching gently combined with breath work, awareness, and relaxation methods, yoga offers a comprehensive approach to increasing flexibility. Using mild positions that enhance flexibility, strength, and balance, we will examine yoga-based stretching techniques appropriate for seniors. Older adults with varying degrees of fitness can do these yoga stretches since they can be tailored to meet individual needs and mobility limitations.

Pilates-Based Stretching:

Pilates is a great kind of exercise for seniors who want to increase their general mobility and function since it has a strong emphasis on core strength, stability, and flexibility. We'll talk about stretching exercises based on Pilates that work on important muscle groups and help you maintain good posture and alignment. These exercises serve to increase joint mobility, strengthen and lengthen muscles, and heighten body awareness.

Stretching methods are crucial to include in your routine if you want to increase your general mobility as a senior reduce stiffness and improve flexibility. You may profit from increased flexibility and move more comfortably and easily in your daily life with regular practice and devotion.

Flexibility Exercises for Different Body Parts

These exercises assist seniors in increasing flexibility, decreasing stiffness, and improving general mobility by concentrating on particular muscle groups and joints. There are exercises made specifically to target your requirements and goals, whether you want to reduce stress in your neck and shoulders, strengthen your hips and lower back, or enhance the range of motion in your legs and ankles. Allow us to explore these flexibility exercises tailored to certain body areas.

Neck and Shoulder Stretches:

In particular, bad posture and extended sitting times can cause seniors to frequently feel tightness and strain in their shoulders and neck. To release tension and increase flexibility in these regions, we'll look at slowly extending the neck, rolling the shoulders, and performing shoulder stretches. By promoting improved alignment and posture, these exercises can assist in reducing pain and improving range of motion.

Spine and Lower Back Stretches:

Seniors who lead sedentary lives or have age-related changes in their spinal health frequently experience stiffness and soreness in the spine and lower back. To increase flexibility and mobility in the spine and lower back, we'll talk about poses like child's pose, sitting spinal twists, and cat-cow stretches. These stretches assist in lengthening the spine, releasing back muscle tension, and enhancing general spinal health.

Hip and Pelvic Stretches:

Seniors who want to preserve their balance, stability, and appropriate gait must have hip mobility. We'll look at hip-opening workouts, piriformis stretches, and hip flexor stretches to increase hip and pelvic range of motion and flexibility. With the help of these exercises, which target tight hip muscles and ease stiffness and hip discomfort, one may move more freely and do tasks more effectively.

Leg and Ankle Stretches:

It might be difficult for seniors to walk, stand, and carry out everyday tasks if they have tightness and stiffness in their legs and ankles. We'll talk about stretches and exercises that improve the flexibility and mobility of the legs and ankles, such as hamstring stretches and ankle circles. These exercises lessen the chance of falling, avoid muscular imbalances, and enhance lower body function in general.

Hand and Wrist Stretches:

To preserve dexterity, grip strength, and hand function in elders, hand and wrist flexibility is needed. The flexibility and mobility of the hands and wrists can be enhanced by doing exercises including finger stretches, wrist rotations, and wrist flexor stretches. Seniors may carry out activities more comfortably and easily thanks to these exercises, which also assist in improving fine motor skills, lessen stiffness, and ease arthritic discomfort.

You must include in your routine flexibility exercises that focus on various body regions to preserve mobility, minimize stiffness, and improve your general well-being as a senior. You may age gracefully and vibrantly and realize your body's full potential with regular practice and commitment.

Flexibility Training Programs for Seniors

Safe and efficient methods of enhancing flexibility, range of motion, and general mobility are the goals of these programs. Seniors may customize their flexibility training to meet specific requirements and goals by combining a range of exercises, strategies, and progressions. This leads us to a detailed examination of the elements of senior flexibility training regimens.

Setting Realistic Goals:

Before beginning a program of flexibility training, seniors should set reasonable objectives based on their desired results and existing levels of flexibility. Setting precise, attainable goals aids in directing the training process and monitoring progress over time, whether the goal is to increase the range of motion in certain joints, lessen stiffness in particular muscle groups, or improve general mobility.

Frequency and Duration:

Seniors who participate in flexibility training programs should have frequent sessions dedicated to mobility and stretching exercises. Spend 20 to 30 minutes a day, at least twice or three times a week, on flexibility exercises as part of your regimen. As you get more accustomed to the exercises, gradually increase the length and intensity of your workouts. Consistency is the key to achieving success, so make an effort to adhere to a routine.

Variety of Exercises:

A comprehensive program of flexibility training ought to incorporate an array of exercises that concentrate on distinct muscle groups and joints across the body. Stretching methods such as static, dynamic, and proprioceptive neuromuscular facilitation (PNF) can be used to increase range of motion and flexibility. To further enhance flexibility, strength, and balance holistically, think about adding yoga, Pilates, or Tai Chi-based workouts.

Warm-Up and Cool-Down:

Seniors need to warm up their muscles and get their bodies ready for movement before beginning any flexibility exercises. Light aerobic exercises like cycling or walking can be used as a gradual warm-up to assist boost blood flow and loosen up muscles. Make sure to incorporate a cool-down phase with light stretching and deep breathing to encourage relaxation and healing after finishing the flexibility exercises.

Progression and Modification:

Over time, seniors can increase the duration and intensity of their workouts to maintain development as they get more accustomed to their flexibility training program. Utilize the concepts of progressive overload by progressively extending the length of stretches, increasing the number of reps, or challenging the exercises. Make sure you adapt the workouts to each person's unique talents and restrictions as well.

Safety and Comfort:

When engaging in flexibility exercise, safety should always come first, especially for older citizens. When performing exercises, focus on using the right form and technique; do not push yourself past your comfort level or cause yourself any discomfort. Before beginning a flexibility training program, see a healthcare provider if you have any current medical ailments or concerns to be sure it's safe and suitable for your requirements.

Seniors may create flexibility training regimens that suit their unique requirements and objectives by establishing reasonable goals, including a range of exercises, and placing a high priority on comfort and safety.

Tips for Safe and Effective Stretching

Stretching is essential for increasing mobility, decreasing the chance of injury, and increasing flexibility, particularly for older adults. To assist seniors, and get the most out of their flexibility training program, we go over some crucial advice for safe and efficient stretching.

Warm-Up Before Stretching:

Seniors must make sure their bodies are warmed up and ready for action before beginning any stretching activities. To improve blood flow to the muscles, raise body temperature, and loosen up joints, spend a short warm-up session doing mild aerobic exercises like walking, cycling, or marching in place. In addition to decreasing the chance of injury, this gets the body ready for stretching.

Start Slowly and Progress Gradually:

Seniors who have never stretched before should start carefully and work their way up to longer and more intense stretches over time. Steer clear of bouncing or jerking motions since they might cause damage or strain to the muscles. As an alternative, concentrate on slow, deliberate stretches and pay attention to your body's cues. Reduce the intensity of the stretch and make adjustments as necessary if you experience any pain or discomfort.

Hold Each Stretch for an Adequate Duration:

Stretches should be held long enough to allow the muscles and connective tissues to progressively lengthen to properly increase flexibility. Try to hold each pose for 15 to 30 seconds while taking deep breaths and letting go of tension. To prevent straining or damaging your muscles, do not overstretch or push yourself beyond your comfort zone. Rather, concentrate on a pleasant stretching sensation and progressively raise the level of difficulty over time.

Focus on Proper Form and Alignment:

For stretching exercises to be as effective as possible and to lower the risk of injury, appropriate form and alignment must be maintained. Make sure you're doing each stretch correctly by paying attention to your posture and body alignment. To give support and stability, contract the muscles around the extended joint; do not lock or overextend your joints.

Breathe Deeply and Relax:

Since it promotes relaxation and relieves muscular tension, deep breathing is a crucial part of a good stretching regimen.

As they prepare for each stretch, seniors should concentrate on breathing deeply and regularly, easing into the pose with calm, deep inhalations and exhaled breaths. As a result, the stretch is more effective, relaxation is encouraged, and stress is decreased.

Stay Hydrated and Well-Nourished:

To maintain flexibility and general musculoskeletal health, one must consume the right foods and beverages. Seniors who stretch should make sure they are properly hydrated before and after since dehydration raises the possibility of injury and cramping in the muscles. Furthermore, keeping up a nutritious, well-balanced diet full of foods high in protein, vitamins, and minerals promotes muscle growth and repair, improving function and flexibility.

Chapter Three
Understanding Balance

In this chapter, we explore the idea of balance and how important it is to seniors' general health and wellbeing. Keeping our balance as we become older is crucial for avoiding falls, retaining our independence, and leading fulfilling lives. Seniors may improve their stability, self-assurance, and mobility by studying the elements that affect balance and investigating methods for achieving better balance. Come with me as we examine the nuances of balance and what it means for seniors.

The Importance of Balance:

The capacity to maintain stability and regulate our body posture throughout a variety of tasks is facilitated by balance, which is a key component of movement and coordination. Being able to balance well is crucial for seniors as falls can result in significant injuries and loss of independence. Seniors who have better balance are more mobile, less likely to fall, and can continue leading active lives long into old age.

Factors Affecting Balance:

Strength in the muscles, flexibility in the joints, vision, proprioception (knowledge of one's body location in space), and vestibular function (inner ear balance) are some of the elements that affect balance. Age-related changes in these parameters, including diminished flexibility, loss of muscle mass, and compromised sensory function, can throw off balance and raise the chance of falling. Comprehending these elements is essential for formulating focused tactics to enhance equilibrium.

Assessing Balance:

To pinpoint areas of weakness and create a training program that effectively addresses balance, it is crucial to first assess balance. Balance may be assessed using a variety of tools, such as the Timed Up and Go Test, Single Leg Stance Test, and Berg Balance Scale. These evaluations support the identification of balancing deficiencies and the monitoring of improvement over time for elders and their healthcare professionals.

Balance Training Exercises:

To improve general balance and lower the risk of falls, balance training activities emphasize strengthening, stabilizing, and coordinating the body. We'll look at many balancing exercises that are appropriate for seniors, such as dynamic balance exercises, weight-shifting activities, and standing balance exercises. Seniors can become more adept at maintaining equilibrium in a variety of scenarios by performing these activities, which test their body's balancing mechanisms.

Tai Chi and Yoga for Balance:

Yoga and tai chi are age-old disciplines that have several advantages for balance, coordination, and general health. We'll talk about how attentive breathing and soft, flowing motions used in Tai Chi and yoga-based workouts may help seniors gain better strength, flexibility, and balance. For seniors with varying degrees of fitness, these activities are advantageous and accessible because they foster body awareness, mindfulness, and relaxation.

Lifestyle Factors:

Several lifestyle choices might impact balance and stability in general in addition to physical activity. For optimum balance and mobility, one must consume enough water, eat a healthy diet, and sleep enough. Apart from eliminating trip risks and making sure their living areas have enough lighting and safety rails, seniors should also be aware of their surroundings.

For seniors who wish to keep their independence, avoid falls, and lead fulfilling lives, they must understand balance. Seniors can increase their stability, self-assurance, and mobility by investigating the elements that affect balance, evaluating balance deficiencies, and putting specific balance training exercises into practice.

Chapter Four
Improving Balance

In this chapter, we discuss methods and drills made especially to help seniors with their balance. Including focused balancing training in a senior's routine can help reduce falls, improve mobility, and support general well-being, since keeping balance becomes more and more vital as they age. Elderly people can benefit from increased stability and self-assurance in their every day activities by comprehending the fundamentals of balance training and putting them into practice with efficient exercises. Let us examine the many methods for enhancing seniors' balance.

Understanding Balance Training:

Proprioception, vestibular function, and neuromuscular coordination are among the balance systems within the body that are tested by balance training exercises and activities. Seniors who consistently engage in targeted workouts that challenge these systems will be better able to manage their body posture and maintain stability during a variety of motions and activities.

Standing Balance Exercises:

Improved stability and control when standing erect are the main goals of standing balancing exercises. Keeping a balance on one leg or uneven surfaces like foam pads or balancing boards is a common task for these workouts. Stand-by-stands, tandem stands, and heel-to-toe stands are a few types of standing balancing exercises. With the use of these exercises, seniors may enhance proprioception, balance control, and lower-body muscular strength.

Weight Shifting Exercises:

Exercises involving weight shifting entail moving the body's weight from side to side or from foot to foot while keeping equilibrium. Seniors can become more adept at adjusting their center of gravity and keeping their stability during dynamic movements by performing these exercises. Exercises that involve moving weight in different directions include diagonal, forward-backward, and side-to-side movements. Balance-related skills like proprioception and coordination are improved by these workouts.

Dynamic Balance Exercises:

Dynamic balancing exercises include motions that test one's ability to maintain balance. Seniors can enhance their capacity to maintain stability when doing functional tasks like walking, ascending stairs, and reaching by engaging in exercises that replicate everyday life activities. Walking heel-to-toe, stepping over obstacles, and walking on uneven terrain are a few examples of dynamic balancing exercises.

These workouts increase general mobility and balance by promoting agility, coordination, and quick reflexes.

Tai Chi and Yoga:

Balance training is included in the soft, flowing motions and mindfulness exercises of tai chi and yoga, two age-old disciplines. These exercises provide relaxation and stress relief while assisting seniors in developing better strength, flexibility, and balance. Whereas yoga places more emphasis on alignment, breath control, and body awareness, tai chi places more emphasis on slow, purposeful motions and changing body weight. Seniors of all fitness levels can practice Tai Chi and yoga, which have several advantages for balance and general well-being.

Incorporating Balance into Daily Activities:

To improve their stability and mobility even more, seniors should include balance training in their regular routines in addition to performing targeted balancing exercises. Simple daily routines like taking frequent walks outside, practicing balance while doing domestic tasks, and brushing your teeth while standing on one leg may all help you become more confident and balanced.

Keeping seniors independent, reducing the risk of falls, and enhancing their general well-being all depend on improving their balance. Seniors can increase their mobility, stability, and self-assurance by using these focused training and activities.

Balance Exercises for Different Body Systems

To improve seniors' general stability and coordination, we will look at balancing exercises in this part that are specially tailored to target various bodily systems. Seniors may enhance their balance and lower their chance of falling by including exercises that test different muscle groups and sensory systems. This will increase their independence and self-assurance in day-to-day activities. Let's take a closer look at balancing exercises that work on various bodily systems.

Proprioceptive Balance Exercises:

The body's capacity to perceive its location and motion in space is known as proprioception. The goal of proprioceptive balancing exercises is to enhance proprioception, which is essential for stability and balance. Exercises for proprioceptive balance include the following examples:

Standing on foam pads or balancing discs is a challenge to proprioception and balance control for seniors who are accustomed to uneven surfaces.

Single-leg balance with eyes closed: Elderly people rely on proprioceptive cues to stay balanced when standing on one leg with their eyes shut.

Tandem stance with head turns: Seniors pose a challenge to proprioception and balance control by standing with one foot immediately in front of the other and rotating their head from side to side.

Vestibular Balance Exercises:

Maintaining balance and spatial orientation is vitally important for the vestibular system, which is housed in the inner ear. Exercises for vestibular balance are designed to activate the vestibular system and enhance stability and balance. Exercises for vestibular balance include the following:

Head movements: The vestibular system is stimulated by seniors moving their heads slowly and deliberately in several directions, such as up, down, left, and right.

Balance while turning: A further challenge to balance regulation and vestibular system function is when seniors tilt their heads side to side while standing on one leg.

Balance on unstable surfaces with head movements: Elderly people test their vestibular system and balance control by standing on foam pads or balancing discs and moving their heads in different directions.

Musculoskeletal Balance Exercises:

Musculoskeletal balance exercises focus on improving strength, flexibility, and coordination in the muscles and joints, which are essential for maintaining balance and stability. Examples of musculoskeletal balance exercises include:

Leg lifts: With a concentration on control and stability, seniors raise one leg off the ground while standing.

Heel-to-toe walk: Seniors enhance their coordination and balance by walking in a straight line, with the heel of one foot always landing in front of the toes of the other.

Squats: To increase lower body strength and stability, seniors focus on correct form and alignment when performing squats while keeping their balance on both feet.

Visual Balance Exercises:

With its ability to provide visual clues about the surroundings, the visual system is vital to the maintenance of balance and spatial orientation. To improve stability and balance, visual balancing exercises emphasize better visual processing and integration. Here are some activities for visual balance:

Seniors can enhance their visual tracking and coordination skills by practicing eye-tracking activities when they track a moving object with their eyes, such as a ball or finger.

Balance with visual distraction: To test their visual processing and integration skills, seniors engage in balancing activities while concentrating on a visual goal, such as a moving or fixed item.

Balance with visual obstruction: To rely on alternative sensory systems, such as proprioception and vestibular input, for balance maintenance, seniors engage in balancing exercises with their eyes closed or while wearing blindfolds.

Balance Training Programs for Seniors

In this section, we investigate thorough balancing training regimens created especially for elderly citizens to increase mobility, decrease the chance of falls, and improve stability. A range of exercises and techniques are incorporated into these programs to address various components of balance, such as proprioception, strength, coordination, and sensory integration. Seniors might gain more confidence in their everyday activities and improve their balance by adhering to systematic balance training programs. Let us examine these programs more thoroughly.

Multicomponent Balance Training:

Strength, flexibility, coordination, proprioception, and other components of balance are all targeted by the many exercises included in multicomponent balance training regimens. To increase general stability and mobility, these programs frequently incorporate weight training, functional movements, and a mix of static and dynamic balancing exercises. Seniors can benefit from multicomponent balance training regimens such as these:

The Otago Exercise Program: The Otago Exercise Program was created especially for senior citizens and includes strength and balance exercises to increase mobility and lower the risk of falls.

The Failproof Balance and Mobility Program: By using a progression of functional motions and exercises, this research-based program aims to improve strength, flexibility, and balance.

The Stepping on Program: To assist seniors in maintaining their independence and lowering their risk of falling, this community-based program offers balancing drills, strength training, and instruction on fall prevention techniques.

Tai Chi and Qigong Programs:

The ancient Chinese martial arts of Tai Chi and Qigong place a strong emphasis on attentive exercises and fluid, gradual motions. Seniors' balance, coordination, and general well-being have all been demonstrated to improve with these exercises. Seniors participating in Tai Chi and Qigong classes usually do a sequence of soft, coordinated motions that test balance and encourage relaxation. Programs that teach Tai Chi and Qigong to older citizens include:

Tai Chi for Arthritis: A set of Tai Chi motions created especially to promote joint health, flexibility, and balance in older adults with arthritis are included in this program, which was created by Dr. Paul Lam.

Tai Ji Quan: Moving for Better Balance: This research-proven program combines a series of Tai Chi exercises and motions to enhance balance and lower the chance of falling.

Group Exercise Classes:

Seniors who take group fitness courses get the chance to participate in regulated balance training programs in a friendly and community setting. Participants in these programs are usually guided through a range of balancing exercises and motions by professional instructors. Senior fitness sessions in groups may consist of:

Balance and stability classes: By using a range of exercises and activities, such as dynamic movements, weight-shifting exercises, and standing balance drills, these programs concentrate on enhancing balance and coordination.

Functional fitness classes: To enhance balance, strength, and mobility, these programs integrate functional motions that resemble everyday tasks like walking, bending, and reaching.

Dance-based classes: Dance-based classes, such as ballet-inspired barre classes or line dancing, offer seniors a fun and engaging way to improve balance, coordination, and flexibility.

Tips for Safe and Effective Balance Training

In this section, we'll go over some crucial advice for seniors looking to practice balance training safely and successfully. An attentive and cautious approach to training is necessary to minimize damage, even though sustaining independence and preventing falls depend heavily on increasing balance. Seniors may improve their balance training regimen and gain greater stability and self-assurance in their every day activities by using the advice in this book.

Start Slowly and Progress Gradually:

Exercise intensity and difficulty should be increased gradually throughout a balanced training program; it is important to start cautiously. Standing on one leg or utilizing unstable surfaces like foam pads or balancing boards are examples of basic balance exercises for seniors to start with. Gradually, seniors should advance to more difficult exercises like standing on both feet or sitting on a solid platform.

Use Proper Form and Alignment:

To reduce the risk of injury and increase the benefits of balancing exercises, it is essential to maintain correct form and alignment. The major goal for seniors should be to keep their shoulders relaxed and their spine in alignment while keeping a tall posture. Place your feet hip-width apart and equally distribute your weight on both feet when doing standing exercises. To stabilize their body and prevent swaying or tilting, elders should also contract their core muscles.

Use Support as Needed:

When doing balancing exercises, seniors should feel comfortable utilizing a chair, countertop, or wall for support, particularly if they are new to the activity or have mobility limitations. Support may progressively develop strength and balance while offering steadiness and confidence. Seniors can gradually rely less on assistance and push themselves with more difficult activities as they become more self-assured and stable.

Focus on Breathing and Relaxation:

Seniors can improve their attention and lower their risk of stress or strain by using deep breathing and relaxation techniques to help them stay calm and focused during balancing training. The emphasis for seniors should be on breathing evenly and deeply—in through the nose and out through the mouth. Seniors can also benefit from practicing relaxation techniques like progressive muscle relaxation or guided imagery, which can help them stay focused and attentive throughout activities.

Incorporate Variety and Progression:

Seniors should include a range of balancing exercises in their program and progressively up the intensity and complexity over time to maintain improved balance and avoid plateaus. Exercises that focus on several facets of balance, such as proprioceptive, dynamic, and static exercises, can be combined to make workouts interesting and difficult. Seniors can also strive to advance their routines as they gain strength and confidence by upping the time, repetitions, or resistance of their workouts.

Listen to Your Body:

The most important thing for seniors to remember while doing balance training is to listen to their bodies and notice any signals of pain. Elderly people should alter or stop doing an activity if it feels too difficult or painful, and they should also seek medical advice if required. To minimize harm and guarantee long-term success in balancing training, it is critical to put safety first and refrain from going over and beyond one's boundaries.

Chapter Five
Integrating Flexibility and Balance

In this chapter, we examine how flexibility and balance work together and how including both in a thorough training program might improve seniors' general mobility, stability, and well-being. Balance and flexibility are strongly connected, and gains in one frequently result in gains in the other. Seniors can benefit from increased joint mobility, better posture, and improved general function by adding flexibility exercises to their balancing training regimen. Let's take a closer look at how to include balance and flexibility workouts.

Understanding the Relationship Between Flexibility and Balance:

While balance is the capacity to remain stable and in balance while engaging in different activities, flexibility is the range of motion surrounding a joint. Because more fluid and controlled motions are possible with increased flexibility, there is a decreased chance of muscular strain and damage, which can help with balance. On the other hand, balancing training can increase joint mobility by encouraging appropriate alignment, posture, and muscle activation, all of which contribute to improved flexibility.

Flexibility Exercises for Balance:

Seniors who participate in balance training programs can benefit from increased joint mobility, less muscular tension, and improved overall movement quality thanks to the inclusion of flexibility exercises. The following are some instances of flexibility exercises that go well with balance training:

Dynamic stretching: Swing your legs, rotate your arms, and twist your body to create gentle, rhythmic movements that stretch your muscles and joints.

Static stretching: For a duration of 15 to 30 seconds, hold mild stretches that target key muscle groups such as the calves, hamstrings, quadriceps, hips, chest, and shoulders.

Yoga poses: Engage in yoga postures including downward dog, forward fold, warrior poses, and sitting spinal twists that focus on coordination and flexibility.

Balance Exercises with Added Flexibility Components:

Further improving joint mobility, stability, and coordination is possible when flexibility components are included in balancing exercises. Exercises for flexibility and balance can help seniors perform better overall and fall less frequently. The following are some instances of balancing exercises that also involve flexibility:

Balance lunges with torso twists: To extend the spine and enhance rotational stability, do lunges while rotating your torso.

Single-leg deadlifts with hamstring stretches: Reach your hands toward your toes during single-leg deadlifts to lengthen your hamstrings and enhance your ability to maintain your balance.

Quadruped hip circles: Improve your hip mobility and stability by balancing on your hands and knees and performing hip circles.

Mind-Body Practices for Flexibility and Balance:

Stress reduction, awareness, and physical health are encouraged by mind-body exercises like Tai Chi, Qigong, and Pilates, which combine elements of flexibility and balance. These techniques, improve general flexibility, balance, and coordination, with an emphasis on deliberate movements, deep breathing, and mental attention. Mind-body exercises are a great way for seniors to increase their general quality of life, decrease stress, and improve joint mobility.

Functional Movement Patterns:

Functional movement patterns are dynamic, multi-joint motions that incorporate elements of flexibility and balance, simulating activities of everyday living. Seniors can enhance their mobility, stability, and coordination in everyday circumstances by engaging in functional movement patterns practice. Here are a few instances of useful movement patterns:

Squat to overhead reach: Enhance your lower body strength, hip mobility, and shoulder flexibility by performing squats with your arms extended overhead.

Step-ups with hip flexor stretch: For better balance, coordination, and hip mobility, actively stretch your hip flexors while performing step-up positions.

Balance ball exercises: To increase your core strength, stability, and general flexibility, try some sitting twists, bridges, and hamstring curls on a balance ball. Seniors can improve their mobility and balance while lowering their risk of falls and injuries by learning how flexibility and balance are related, and by incorporating a range of exercises such as dynamic and static stretching, yoga poses, mind-body techniques, and functional movement patterns.

Strategies for Maintaining Flexibility and Balance Over Time

We will explore key tactics that older adults may use to maintain their flexibility and balance throughout time. While increasing balance and flexibility is important, preserving these traits calls for constant work and close attention to detail. Seniors may ensure continued growth and lower their risk of falls and mobility problems by putting these techniques into practice and incorporating them into their everyday lives. Let's take a closer look at these tactics.

Consistent Practice:

For flexibility and balance to last over time, consistency is essential. Even on days when they may not feel like it, seniors should make an effort to include flexibility and balance exercises in their regular regimen. Seniors can experience ongoing improvements in their mobility and stability by creating and adhering to a regular practice routine that will help them form enduring habits.

Gradual Progression:

Seniors should take their time while starting flexibility and balance exercises, just like with any other physical activity. Accidents and setbacks might result from pushing too hard or moving too fast. To enable their bodies to adjust and strengthen healthily, seniors should instead progressively increase the volume, duration, or complexity of their workouts over time.

Variety in Exercises:

Seniors should mix up their regimen with a range of flexibility and balancing exercises to avoid boredom and plateaus. Workouts may remain interesting and demanding by varying the exercises that focus on various muscle groups and movement patterns. Variety also makes sure that every facet of flexibility and balance is taken care of, which results in more thorough gains.

Mindful Movement:

By encouraging awareness of the body and its motions, mindfulness practices can improve the efficacy of training in flexibility and balance. Moving attentively and paying attention to alignment, breath, and body sensations should be the main focus for seniors. Moving with awareness not only increases physical performance but also lowers stress and promotes general wellbeing.

Functional Training:

To integrate flexibility and balance elements into useful movements, functional training focuses on exercises that replicate activities of everyday living. Seniors' capacity to carry out daily duties safely and effectively can be enhanced by engaging in regular functional exercise. To further promote general functional independence, functional exercise also improves joint stability and mobility.

Regular Assessment:

It is crucial to regularly evaluate balance and flexibility to monitor development and pinpoint areas that still require work. To determine their overall level of fitness, seniors should routinely assess their functional mobility, balance, and range of motion. To address certain shortcomings or imbalances, the training program may be modified in light of the evaluation results.

Injury Prevention:

Over time, preserving flexibility and balance requires preventing injuries. To prepare the body and avoid muscular strains or injuries, seniors should place a high priority on following appropriate warm-up and cool-down protocols both before and after exercise sessions. Seniors should also pay attention to their bodies and refrain from overdoing it or working through discomfort when exercising.

Lifestyle Factors:

Maintaining flexibility and balance is greatly influenced by lifestyle choices including diet, hydration, sleep patterns, and stress reduction. Seniors should place a high priority on eating a well-balanced, nutrient-dense diet, drinking enough water, getting enough sleep, and engaging in stress-relieving activities like relaxation or meditation. These lifestyle choices promote general health and ideal bodily function. Maintaining flexibility and balance requires a combination of elements such as regular evaluation, injury avoidance, conscious movement, functional training, varied exercise regimens, steady practice, and lifestyle choices.

Chapter Six
Overcoming Common Challenges

This chapter discusses typical obstacles that seniors may run across when trying to increase their balance and flexibility, as well as solutions for them. Seniors must overcome obstacles ranging from physical constraints to psychological barriers to reach their fitness objectives and preserve their independence in day-to-day living. Let's examine these issues in more detail and talk about practical solutions for each.

Dealing with the Fear of Falling

One of the most common concerns among seniors is fear of falling, which can hurt their self-esteem and willingness to participate in stretching and balance-enhancing exercises. In this chapter, we'll look at methods for dealing with and getting over the fear of falling, which will help seniors feel more secure and independent in their everyday lives.

Education and Awareness:

Increasing awareness and educating yourself is one of the best strategies to get over your fear of falling. Seniors might benefit from knowing the typical reasons why people fall, the effects of falling, and doable preventative measures. Seniors who have more knowledge at their disposal may feel more capable and self-assured when it comes to controlling their fear.

Fall Prevention Strategies:

Fall risk can be decreased and seniors' sense of security in their surroundings increased by putting fall prevention methods into practice. Making little but effective changes to the house, such as reducing trip hazards, adding grab bars to the bathroom, and upgrading the lighting, may have a big impact on encouraging safety and comfort.

Strength and Balance Training:

Seniors who regularly engage in strength and balance training activities might lessen their fear of falling and develop a greater sense of confidence in their physical capabilities. Seniors can become more adept and confident in their abilities to do everyday tasks by increasing their physical strength, coordination, and stability.

Gradual Exposure:

Seniors might become less sensitive to the fear of falling and gradually gain confidence by gradually exposing them to fear-inducing activities. Seniors can begin by working on their balance in a safe, supported atmosphere. As they get more secure and comfortable, they can work their way up to increasingly difficult exercises.

Mindfulness and Relaxation Techniques:

Seniors who struggle with anxiety can learn mindfulness and relaxation techniques including progressive muscle relaxation, deep breathing, and meditation. These skills can also help them feel less afraid of falling. Seniors can face difficult situations with increased confidence and clarity of mind by practicing presence and serenity.

Support and Social Connection:

Seniors who are trying to get over their fear of falling may find comfort and encouragement in asking for help from friends, family, or support organizations. Seniors can develop a feeling of community and camaraderie by interacting with people who have gone through similar things. This helps them remember that they are not traveling alone.

Professional Guidance:

Healthcare specialists who specialize in fall prevention and rehabilitation, such as occupational therapists or physical therapists, may be able to provide important help to seniors who experience a fear of falling. These experts are capable of doing risk factor assessments, making customized recommendations, and delivering treatments that are specifically designed to address issues that may arise.

Positive Self-Talk and Affirmations:

Seniors who are encouraged to counter negative attitudes with more empowered thoughts and beliefs might benefit from positive self-talk and affirmations. Seniors may develop a mindset of resilience, strength, and confidence in their abilities to overcome problems by rephrasing frightening ideas into uplifting affirmations.

Addressing Pain and Discomfort

One typical obstacle that seniors may face while trying to increase their flexibility and balance is pain and discomfort. Chronic pain can have a major negative influence on motivation, mobility, and general quality of life. This chapter covers pain and discomfort management techniques that help seniors get beyond setbacks and keep moving in the direction of increased flexibility and balance.

Consultation with Healthcare Professionals:

Seniors should always seek advice from medical specialists, such as doctors, physical therapists, or chiropractors when they are in pain or uncomfortable. This will help to determine the root cause of the issue and create a customized treatment plan. To successfully manage pain and discomfort, healthcare experts can do evaluations, identify certain diseases, and suggest suitable therapies.

Proper Warm-up and Cool-down:

Seniors should complete a suitable warm-up regimen to get their bodies ready for physical activity before beginning flexibility and balancing exercises. Light cardiovascular, dynamic stretching and mobility exercises are all important components of a warm-up since they improve blood flow, relax muscles, and lower the chance of injury. Static stretching and relaxation methods can also be used as part of a cool-down regimen to assist avoid stiffness in the muscles and speed up recovery after physical activity.

Modification of Exercises:

Exercise modifications are recommended for seniors who are in pain or uncomfortable so they may continue to be physically active without aggravating their symptoms. A few examples of modifications are limiting the range of motion, changing the duration or intensity of workouts, or selecting fewer taxing alternatives that are easier on the body. Seniors must pay attention to their bodies and refrain from pushing through discomfort since doing so might result in more harm.

Incorporation of Low-impact Activities:

Seniors may maintain an active lifestyle while lowering joint stress pain and discomfort by engaging in low-impact sports like swimming, cycling, or water aerobics. For seniors with chronic pain or mobility concerns, these activities are appropriate because they provide the advantages of cardiovascular exercise without unduly taxing the muscles and joints.

Application of Heat and Cold Therapy:

Joint stiffness, inflammation, and muscular soreness can all be treated with heat and cold treatment to reduce pain and suffering. Seniors who have aching muscles or joints might enhance blood flow and induce relaxation by applying heat packs, warm compresses, or heating pads. Cold treatment, which includes applying ice packs or cold compresses to the afflicted region, can also help lower inflammation and dull discomfort.

Mind-body Techniques:

Through the promotion of relaxation, reduction of stress, and enhancement of general well-being, mind-body therapies including progressive muscle relaxation, guided imagery, deep breathing, and meditation can assist seniors in managing pain and discomfort. Seniors may manage their discomfort and have a positive view of their health and rehabilitation by implementing these tactics into their everyday routines.

Medication Management:

To reduce symptoms and enhance quality of life, seniors who are in chronic pain may need to have their medications managed. Together with their healthcare practitioners, seniors should create a personalized drug plan that minimizes any possible adverse effects or interactions while meeting their individual needs. It is crucial that elderly patients take their medications as directed and let their doctor know if their symptoms change or cause them to have concerns.

Psychological Support:

Feelings of irritation, worry, or sadness can result from chronic pain, which can have a substantial psychological impact. To treat mental anguish and create coping mechanisms for pain management, seniors may find it helpful to receive psychological support through counseling or support groups. Creating a solid support system of friends, family, and medical experts may provide seniors the motivation and direction they need to go through their path toward pain management and better health.

Chapter Seven
Lifestyle Factors for Flexibility and Balance

A person's flexibility and balance are mostly determined by their lifestyle choices. Everyday activities can have an influence on one's physical capabilities and general well-being, from proper diet and water to stress reduction and sleep hygiene. To promote seniors' maximum mobility and stability, we examine the significance of lifestyle variables for flexibility and balance in this chapter and offer doable methods for maximizing these aspects.

Nutrition and Hydration:

Staying hydrated and eating a healthy diet is crucial for maintaining balance and flexibility. To ensure that their muscles and joints receive the nutrition they need, seniors should strive for a balanced diet full of fruits, vegetables, lean meats, whole grains, and healthy fats. In addition, maintaining proper tissue hydration and supporting overall physical performance may be achieved by drinking enough water throughout the day.

Sleep Quality:

To retain flexibility and balance, muscles must develop, heal, and recover from injuries. All of these processes depend on getting enough sleep. In addition to practicing appropriate sleep hygiene practices, which include adhering to a regular sleep schedule, setting up a calming bedtime ritual, and maximizing the comfort and relaxation of their sleeping environment, seniors should place a high priority on receiving adequate sleep every night.

Physical Activity:

To keep your flexibility, strength, and balance, you must exercise regularly. Stretching, balancing, weight training, and cardiovascular activity are just a few of the activities seniors should partake in to improve their mobility, stability, and coordination. Different forms of physical activity incorporated into everyday activities can help seniors become more fit overall and lower their chance of injury and falls.

Stress Management:

Extended periods of stress can exacerbate tense muscles, impede coordination and focus, and severely affect flexibility and balance. To promote relaxation, reduce tension, and enhance mental clarity, seniors can benefit from practicing stress management practices including yoga, tai chi, meditation, and deep breathing. Other ways to reduce stress and enhance general wellbeing include taking part in pleasant activities, going outside, and spending time with loved ones.

Posture and Body Mechanics:

It is crucial to maintain proper body mechanics and posture to avoid musculoskeletal problems, maintain flexibility, and maintain balance. Seniors should be aware of their posture at all times, especially when sitting or standing for extended periods. They should also try to prevent slouching or hunching over. Using good body mechanics when performing routine tasks like bending over or lifting goods can help lower the chance of straining or injuring your muscles and joints.

Cognitive Health:

Since cognitive function motor abilities and coordination are intimately related, cognitive health is important for maintaining flexibility and balance. To maintain mental health and improve general physical performance, seniors should take part in cognitively demanding activities like games, puzzles, and learning new skills. Furthermore, upholding social ties and engaging in mental stimulation can enhance cognitive performance and enhance general quality of life.

Environmental Factors:

Flexibility and balance in older adults can be impacted by environmental variables, such as home safety and accessibility. By removing trip hazards, adding handrails and grab bars, and making sure the entire house has enough lighting, seniors can make it a safe and encouraging place to be. To avoid slipping, tripping, and falling, seniors should also be aware of the surface conditions and the weather when they are outside.

Nutrition and Hydration Tips

Being well-nourished and hydrated is critical for preserving flexibility and balance because it gives the body the nutrients and fluids it needs for healthy joints and muscles. To foster flexibility and balance, we look at some doable advice and suggestions in this chapter for seniors on how to improve their eating and drinking habits.

Balanced Diet:

Flexibility and balance are supported best by a varied, well-balanced diet full of nutrients. A wide variety of foods should be a goal for seniors' diets, with an emphasis on:

Fruits and vegetables: To include vital vitamins, minerals, and antioxidants that promote the health of your muscles and joints, include a colorful assortment of fruits and vegetables in your meals and snacks.

Lean proteins: To promote muscle growth and repair, go for lean protein sources including fish, chicken, beans, lentils, tofu, and low-fat dairy.

Whole grains: Make room for whole grains, which include quinoa, brown rice, oats, and whole wheat bread. These foods include fiber to support digestive health and complex carbs for long-lasting energy.

Healthy fats: Add foods high in healthy fats, such as avocados, almonds, seeds, and olive oil, to help lubricate joints and lower inflammation.

Adequate Hydration:

To prevent weariness, cramping in the muscles, and decreased physical performance, it is essential to be well-hydrated to preserve balance and flexibility. In warmer weather, after activity, and during illness, seniors should make it a point to stay hydrated throughout the day. Pale yellow urine indicates sufficient hydration; thus, elders can monitor the color of their pee to determine their level of hydration.

Timing of Meals and Snacks:

Meal and snack timing can affect digestion, physical performance, and energy levels. Seniors should make an effort to have frequent, well-balanced meals and snacks throughout the day to keep their blood sugar levels constant and provide their muscles and joints with a consistent supply of energy. At every meal, consuming a mix of healthy fats, proteins, and carbs can enhance overall well-being and maximize the absorption of nutrients.

Pre- and Post-Exercise Nutrition:

To maximize flexibility and balance, support muscle recovery, and fuel exercises, a proper diet is crucial both before and after exercise. Before working out, seniors should have a balanced breakfast or snack that includes both protein and carbs to help muscle regeneration and give them energy. Seniors who exercise should replace their glycogen levels and speed up muscle recovery by refueling with a combination of carbs and protein.

Nutrient-Rich Foods for Flexibility and Balance:

Regular consumption of the following nutrients is recommended since they are essential for maintaining flexibility and balance in the diet:

Omega-3 fatty acids: Omega-3 fatty acids are included in walnuts, chia seeds, flaxseeds, and fatty seafood. They enhance joint health by lowering inflammation.

Calcium and vitamin D: Diets high in calcium, such as dairy products, leafy greens, and fortified meals, and high in vitamin D, like fatty fish, eggs, and fortified dairy products, maintain healthy bones and lower the incidence of fractures.

Antioxidants: Antioxidants, which enhance general joint health and mobility, may be found in fruits, vegetables, nuts, and seeds. They also help minimize oxidative stress and inflammation.

Importance of Sleep for Recovery

Flexibility and balance are only two aspects of general health and well-being that are greatly aided by sleep. Sufficient sleep is necessary for healthy muscular growth, recuperation, and repair in addition to maintaining mental and emotional clarity. To improve flexibility and balance, we discuss the significance of sleep for seniors and offer helpful advice on how to improve their sleep patterns in this chapter.

Muscle Repair and Regeneration:

The body goes through vital regeneration and repair activities as you sleep, including the development and repair of muscular tissue. The body uses sleep to repair injured muscle fibers, restore energy reserves, and flush out metabolic waste products that are collected during the day. Maintaining flexibility and balance as well as promoting the best possible muscle recovery depends on getting enough sleep, both in terms of quantity and quality.

Hormonal Regulation:

Hormones influencing metabolism, muscle development, and repair are largely regulated by sleep. Development hormone supports muscle development and repair, aiding in the recovery process after exercise and encouraging muscle regeneration. It is mostly released during deep sleep periods. Furthermore, getting enough sleep aids in the regulation of cortisol levels, a stress hormone that, when increased, can hinder muscle regeneration and repair.

Cognitive Function:

Restoring memories, acquiring new information, and making decisions all depend on getting enough sleep. Sustaining balance and mobility requires improved cognitive function, response time, and coordination, all of which are enhanced by getting enough sleep, both in terms of quantity and quality. Seniors who don't get enough sleep may be more vulnerable to cognitive decline and worse physical function.

Immune Function:

The immune system and general health are greatly aided by getting enough sleep. To combat infection and control inflammation, the immune system produces proteins known as cytokines while you sleep. Getting enough sleep lowers the chance of being sick and infected and boosts the immune system's defense against pollutants. Elderly people who make sleep a priority can strengthen their defenses against disease and trauma.

Emotional Well-being:

Emotional control and mental wellness depend on getting enough sleep. Sufficient sleep in terms of both length and quality elevates mood, lowers stress levels, and strengthens resistance to emotional difficulties. Seniors who struggle with sleep difficulties or sleep deprivation may be more susceptible to mood disorders like anxiety and depression, which can impair their quality of life and physical functioning.

Practical Tips for Optimizing Sleep:

Create a regular sleep schedule by going to bed and waking up at the same time every day, including on the weekends, to help your body's internal clock function properly and encourage deep sleep.

Create a Relaxing Bedtime Routine: Establishing a calming evening ritual might help your body recognize when it's time to wind down and get ready for sleep. Exercises like reading, light stretching, or using relaxation techniques may fall under this category.

Create a Sleep-Friendly Environment: Maintain a cold, dark, and quiet environment in your bedroom to promote sleep. Invest in a comfy mattress and pillows, and think about utilizing white noise machines or earplugs to drown out annoying noise.

Limit Stimulants and Electronics: Nicotine and coffee should be avoided right before bed since they might disrupt your sleep. Limit your time spent in front of screens and other electronics as well since the blue light they create might interfere with your sleep.

Manage Stress and Anxiety: Before going to bed, try some stress-reduction exercises like progressive muscle relaxation, deep breathing, or meditation to help you relax and quiet your thoughts.

Exercise Regularly: Maintain a regular exercise schedule, but steer clear of intense workouts just before bed since they may be stimulating and disrupt sleep. For your body to have time to relax, try to wrap up your workout at least a couple of hours before bed.

Stress Management Techniques

Everyday living frequently involves stress, which can negatively affect one's flexibility and balance as well as one's physical and mental health. Prolonged stress can impair cognitive function, cause reduced mobility, tense muscles, and damage one's ability to maintain stability and balance. To lower stress levels and promote flexibility and balance, seniors can benefit from implementing the many stress management approaches we discuss in this chapter.

Deep Breathing Exercises:

One easy and efficient technique to lower tension and encourage relaxation is to practice deep breathing. Seniors may learn to breathe deeply by gently exhaling through their lips after taking a deep breath with their noses and letting their bellies expand. They should concentrate on letting go of stress with each breath. You may easily generate a sense of peace and relaxation with deep breathing techniques, which you can practice anywhere, at any time.

Progressive Muscle Relaxation (PMR):

The goal of progressive muscle relaxation is to ease tension and promote relaxation by gradually tensing and releasing the body's various muscle groups. Seniors may begin by tensing certain muscular groups, such as the shoulders, hands, arms, and legs, for a brief period. Afterward, they may release the tension and let the muscles fully relax. Seniors can improve their awareness of muscular tension and their ability to release it by frequently engaging in PMR exercises.

Mindfulness Meditation:

Seniors can develop a sense of peace and alertness by practicing mindfulness meditation, which is concentrating attention on the current moment without passing judgment. Seniors who are interested in mindfulness meditation can do so by finding a peaceful place to sit and paying attention to their thoughts, feelings, and experiences without becoming sucked into them. It has been demonstrated that practicing mindfulness meditation may lower stress, elevate mood, and improve general well-being.

Yoga and Tai Chi:

Together with physical postures, breathing exercises, and meditation, yoga, and tai chi are mild mind-body activities that help people unwind and manage stress. Elderly people can enhance their strength, flexibility, and balance while cultivating a calm and peaceful attitude via yoga and tai chi. Seniors looking for a practice that fits their requirements and tastes can select from a wide range of yoga and tai chi techniques.

Guided Imagery:

With the help of guided imagery, one may visualize serene and relaxing situations or experiences to aid in stress relief and relaxation. Seniors who want to de-stress might make their visualizations or listen to recordings of guided imagery. Seniors can induce emotions of calm and inner peace, which lower stress and improve general well-being, by visualizing themselves in a serene environment, such as a beach or forest.

Engaging in Relaxing Activities:

It is possible to assist elders manage stress and enhance their general mood and well-being by getting them involved in activities that encourage fun and relaxation. To decompress and rejuvenate, seniors might take up activities like painting, gardening, relaxing in nature, or listening to music. Choosing enjoyable and fulfilling hobbies can encourage seniors' efforts to become more flexible and balanced as well as help them handle stress more successfully.

Social Support:

Seniors can receive emotional support and encouragement during stressful times by staying involved in social activities and asking friends, family, or support groups for help. Elderly people can seek support and assistance, get affirmation and understanding, and talk about their thoughts and experiences with someone they can trust. The ability to manage stress and enhance resilience and general well-being in seniors can be achieved by creating a robust support system.

Other Lifestyle Factors Impacting Flexibility and Balance

Aside from diet, hydration, sleep, and stress reduction, several additional elements of everyday living can have an impact on one's physical health and ability to retain flexibility and balance. In this chapter, we examine other lifestyle elements that affect balance and flexibility and provide seniors with doable tactics to maximize these aspects to enhance their general well-being and mobility.

Physical Activity Levels:

Maintaining balance, strength, and flexibility requires regular physical exercise. Seniors should try to include a range of exercises in their program, such as cardiovascular, strength, flexibility, and balance training. Seniors can lower their chances of falls and injuries and increase their general level of fitness by participating in regular physical exercise.

Posture and Body Mechanics:

Maintaining flexibility and balance as well as avoiding musculoskeletal problems needs good posture and body mechanics. Over the day, seniors should be aware of their posture and try to prevent slouching or hunching over, particularly when sitting or standing for extended periods. When doing regular tasks like lifting things or bending over, using good body mechanics can help lower the chance of strain or damage to the muscles and joints.

Environmental Factors:

Flexibility and balance in older adults can be impacted by environmental variables, such as home safety and accessibility. By removing trip hazards, adding handrails and grab bars, and making sure the entire house has enough lighting, seniors can make it a safe and encouraging place to be. To avoid slipping, tripping, and falling, seniors should also be aware of the surface conditions and the weather when they are outside.

Medication Management:

Certain drugs may have a direct or indirect impact on a person's ability to move, balance, and stretch. Seniors should talk to their healthcare practitioner about any concerns they may have and be aware of the possible negative effects of the drugs they take. To provide the best possible management of chronic illnesses while reducing the risk of negative effects on physical function, patients must adhere to the rules for taking their prescription medications and notify healthcare professionals of any changes in symptoms.

Social Connections:

Retaining social ties and remaining involved in the community helps improve balance and flexibility. Seniors who engage in volunteer work, social activities, or community events are more likely to maintain mental and physical stimulation, which lowers the risk of social isolation and enhances general well-being. Developing strong social ties can help one feel motivated, emotionally supported, and encouraged to maintain an active and healthy lifestyle.

Mental Well-being:

Physical mobility and health are strongly correlated with mental well-being. A higher risk of physical decline and decreased flexibility and balance may be faced by seniors who suffer from anxiety, depression, or other mental health concerns. Seniors must put their mental health first by engaging in stress-reduction strategies, seeing mental health specialists for help, and participating in enjoyable and relaxing activities.

Seniors can take proactive measures to enhance their physical well-being and improve their general health and mobility by taking into account certain lifestyle variables that affect flexibility and balance.

Chapter Eight
Real-Life Success Stories

In this chapter, we explore the true success stories of people who have surmounted flexibility and balance-related obstacles. Seniors who may be embarking on their path to enhance their physical well-being might get inspiration and encouragement from these stories. By telling these tales, we hope to demonstrate the strength of tenacity, persistence, and resolve in obtaining more adaptability and balance in daily life.

Sarah's Journey to Improved Balance:

Sarah, a retired schoolteacher, has balance problems as a result of aging and a past knee injury. Sarah signed up for balance training sessions at her neighborhood community center because she was determined to restore her stability and confidence. Through focused workouts and repetition, Sarah steadily increased her balance with the help of her peers and teacher. Sarah is happy to say that she can now walk confidently without worrying about falling and that she now likes engaging in things that she used to shun.

Tom's Transformation Through Yoga:

Tom, a retired accountant, had arthritis and years of sedentary job that left him stiff and with little flexibility.

Tom, in search of solace, chose to give yoga a try after learning about its advantages for stress alleviation and joint mobility. Tom committed to practicing yoga daily despite his initial reservations, and he quickly saw gains in his flexibility, balance, and general well-being. Tom saw improvements in his body's flexibility, agility, and sense of calm with each session. Tom still does yoga daily now and urges others to discover the healing potential of this age-old discipline.

Maria's Recovery from Injury:

Maria, who has always danced, experienced a setback when she sustained a hip injury that limited her range of motion and prevented her from engaging in her favorite pastimes. Maria started a recovery program that included physical therapy, mild exercise, and patience because she was determined to restore her strength and mobility. Maria was able to progressively restore her flexibility, balance, and confidence with persistent work and devotion. Her fortitude and upbeat demeanor served as an example to others around her of the strength of tenacity in the face of difficulty.

Jack's Journey to Active Aging:

Jack, a retired engineer, embraced an active lifestyle in his senior years, participating in activities such as hiking, cycling, and gardening. However, as he aged, Jack began to notice a decline in his flexibility and balance, making it challenging to enjoy his favorite hobbies. Refusing to let age slow him down, Jack sought guidance from fitness professionals and incorporated targeted exercises into his routine to improve his flexibility and balance. With determination and consistency, Jack regained his mobility and continued to lead an active and fulfilling life well into his golden years.

These true success stories show how commitment, tenacity, and fortitude can make a big difference when it comes to conquering obstacles with flexibility and balance. People have discovered methods to enhance their physical well-being and restore their independence and vigor, whether via specialized workouts, alternative treatments, or rehabilitation programs. Our goal is to motivate and encourage seniors to take the first step toward improved flexibility, balance, and general well-being by sharing these motivational tales.

Stories of Seniors Who Improved Flexibility and Balance

We will examine the real-world achievements of elderly people who have significantly increased their flexibility and balance. These motivational stories highlight people's tenacity, fortitude, and resiliency as they overcome obstacles and improve their physical well-being. Our goal in sharing these tales with readers is to inspire and enable them to set out on their path toward better balance and flexibility as they approach senior year.

Martha's Journey to Enhanced Flexibility:

Martha was a late 60s retiree who suffered from arthritis and a sedentary lifestyle that caused her to be stiff and limited in her movement. Martha started going to yoga sessions at her neighborhood community center because she was determined to restore her flexibility and mobility. Martha persisted in her practice, adjusting her postures and moderate stretches to suit her requirements despite some initial difficulties. Martha saw notable gains in her range of motion, flexibility, and general well-being over time. Martha still does yoga daily now and appreciates the increased freedom and energy it gives her.

John's Transformation Through Tai Chi:

Due to his advanced age and history of falls, John, a veteran in his 70s, experienced balance problems and muscular weakness. John turned to tai chi, a martial art renowned for its slow, flowing motions and emphasis on balance and stability, as a gentle yet effective technique to enhance his coordination and balance. John practiced tai chi every day at home and in lessons, showing commitment and regularity.

This helped him build stronger muscles, correct posture, and improve his balance overall. John shares his enthusiasm for this age-old discipline and its life-changing effects with other elders in his community by teaching tai chi sessions, having been inspired by his development.

Alice's Recovery from Injury:

Alice was a retired nurse in her early seventies who had a setback when she fell and damaged her hip. Alice underwent surgery and started a strenuous rehabilitation program aimed at strengthening her muscles and enhancing her balance because she was determined to restore her mobility and independence. Alice steadily improved, progressively recovering her flexibility, balance, and confidence with the help of her family and her medical team. Alice is glad for the chance to resume her active lifestyle and is enjoying hobbies like walking, gardening, and dancing now that she is back on her feet.

George's Active Lifestyle in Retirement:

In his 80s, George was still an athlete, and he didn't let becoming older stop him. George persevered in his commitment to being active and preserving his flexibility and balance despite obstacles like arthritis and joint discomfort. To maintain his muscles strong and his joints supple, he included a range of exercises in his program, such as swimming, cycling, and strength training. George maintains an active lifestyle by pushing himself and encouraging others to enjoy the benefits of physical activity even in their older years. He does this by participating in local sporting activities and maintaining a positive outlook.

Testimonials and Insights from Participants

We examine the testimonies and observations of people who have taken part in projects or programs designed to increase balance and flexibility. These first-hand reports and insightful viewpoints illuminate the difficulties, victories, and lessons discovered on the path to improved physical well-being. Inspiring and motivating readers to look for ways to improve their flexibility and balance is our goal in sharing these testimonies.

Mark's Testimonial: **Finding Strength and Stability Through Yoga**

Mark, an early 70s retiree, talks about how he improved his flexibility and balance by practicing yoga and how it changed his life. Following years of living a sedentary lifestyle, Mark began to experience stiffness and soreness in his muscles and joints, which made it challenging to carry out everyday tasks. He heard about the advantages of yoga for stress alleviation and mobility, so in search of some solace, he gave it a shot. Though at first uneasy, Mark quickly came to love the exercise, progressively developing balance, strength, and flexibility with each session. Mark had a long-overdue sense of serenity and calm in addition to an improvement in his physical health as a result of his persistent hard work and devotion.

Insight: Mark stresses that to benefit from yoga, one must be persistent and patient. He exhorts people to embrace the practice with an open mind and a readiness to discover what their bodies are capable of, believing that practice and patience would bring improvement.

Susan's Insight: Overcoming Fear of Falling Through Tai Chi

Senior Susan, who is in her late 60s, talks about how she used tai chi to help her overcome anxiety and uncertainty. Susan decided to sign up for a tai chi class to strengthen her balance and coordination after suffering a fall that made her feel exposed and uneasy. She was at first apprehensive but eventually found comfort in the soft, flowing motions of tai chi, which helped her gain steadiness, strength, and self-assurance. Susan overcame her fear of falling and restored her sense of empowerment by learning to believe in her body's capacity to move elegantly and purposefully with the help of her instructor and the support of her classmates.

Insight: Susan emphasizes the value of support systems and the community in overcoming obstacles about balance and flexibility. Seeing the benefits of shared experiences and objectives for general well-being, she exhorts elders to look for chances for social interaction and support from one another.

***David's Testimonial*: Embracing a New Lease on Life Through Strength Training**

David, a retired man in his late 70s, talks about how a committed strength training program helped him regain his power and energy. David decided to take control of his health and fitness by adding regular strength training workouts into his regimen after seeing a reduction in muscle mass and mobility. David surprised himself with his newfound talents as he progressively rebuilt strength, flexibility, and balance with the help of a personal trainer and a dedication to consistency. David leads an active lifestyle these days, engaging in sports like cycling, hiking, and gardening with confidence and ease.

Insight: David stresses the need to have reasonable objectives and acknowledge minor accomplishments along the road. He advises elders to approach strength training with endurance and patience, understanding that gains may be slow but eventually fruitful in terms of their total physical health.

Lessons Learned and Inspirational Messages

This chapter offers us a chance to consider the motivational messages and life lessons that may be drawn from the experiences of actual people who have become more flexible and balanced. For readers embarking on their road toward improved physical well-being, these insights provide insightful advice and inspiration. Our goal is to encourage and enable readers to face obstacles head-on, welcome change, and work toward improved health and vitality as they age. We accomplish this by sharing the knowledge and experiences of others.

Embracing Resilience:

The significance of perseverance in the face of difficulty is a recurrent topic in the success tales. Many people had to overcome hardships like disease, injury, or a fear of falling, but they didn't let these things define who they were. Rather, they adopted resilience, converting failures into chances for development and education. Their experiences serve as a reminder that overcoming obstacles head-on with bravery and tenacity is what resilience is all about, not avoiding them.

Celebrating Progress:

The success tales also teach us the value of acknowledging and appreciating any achievement, no matter how tiny. Many people saw progressive gains in their balance and flexibility over time, frequently as a result of persistent hard work and devotion. Through the process of recognizing and commemorating every significant achievement, they maintained their drive and inspiration to pursue their quest for improved physical health. Their experiences serve as a reminder that development is not always linear and that each accomplishment should be welcomed.

Cultivating Mindfulness:

A common practice among many of the people who were successful in increasing their balance and flexibility turned out to be mindfulness. They learned to build awareness of their body, breath, and mind via mindful movement techniques such as yoga, tai chi, or other forms of exercise. They were able to lower stress levels, improve their general well-being, and pay attention to their bodies' demands thanks to their increased awareness. Their experiences demonstrate the transforming potential of mindfulness in promoting a stronger sense of peace and connectedness within oneself.

Seeking Support:

One common element across the success tales is how crucial it is to ask for help when you need it. On their path to greater flexibility and balance, many people found strength and encouragement in the assistance of others, whether from peers, teachers, or medical experts. Being surrounded by a network of support gave them the confidence to conquer obstacles, maintain motivation, and endure tough trying times. Their experiences highlight the importance of relationships and teamwork in accomplishing common objectives.

Embracing Possibilities:

The success tales' most motivational lesson may be to always remember that it's never too late to become more flexible and balanced. Every person discovered a way ahead toward improved health and vitality, regardless of age or physical state. Their tales demonstrate the human spirit's tenacity and the limitless possibilities for development and change, even in the latter years of life. Their experiences encourage us to seize fresh opportunities, take calculated chances, and bravely and resolutely follow our passions.

For readers on their journey toward greater flexibility and balance, the real-life success stories presented in this chapter provide insightful insights and motivational messages. Many people have seen incredible improvements in their physical well-being through perseverance, celebration, awareness, support, and an openness to new opportunities.

Conclusion
Embracing Flexibility and Balance in the Senior Years

As we get to the end of "Flexibility and Balance for Seniors," it's important to take a moment to digest the main ideas that were covered in this book. We should also think about the recommendations and parting words of wisdom that will help us reach our goals of improved physical health as we age.

Concepts Explored:

This book has covered a lot of ground about how flexibility and balance help us stay mobile, independent, and healthy as we age. We have discussed how our flexibility, stability, and general quality of life might be affected by the physiological changes that the body experiences throughout time. The advantages of consistent exercise, mindfulness training, and lifestyle adjustments in strengthening flexibility, boosting balance, and lowering the risk of falls and injuries have been demonstrated. Also, we've spoken about how to maintain our physical well-being and maximize our flexibility and balance through proper diet, hydration, sleep, and stress management.

Action Plans:

Now that we have this information, it is time to apply what we have learned. To improve our balance and flexibility in our senior years, we should think about the following action plans:

Create an exercise regimen that is specific to you that incorporates aerobic, strength, flexibility, and balance training.

Incorporate mindfulness exercises to encourage relaxation, lower stress levels, and enhance bodily awareness, such as yoga, tai chi, or meditation, into your everyday routine. Make eating a balanced diet full of fruits, vegetables, lean meats, whole grains, and healthy fats a priority. You should also drink enough water to keep hydrated throughout the day. Take steps to make your house secure and encouraging by removing any potential dangers, adding grab bars and handrails, and making sure there is enough lighting. Consult with medical experts, personal trainers, and neighborhood resources to create a customized strategy that fits your requirements and objectives.

Final Words of Wisdom:

These last bits of wisdom should be kept in mind as we go out on our path toward more flexibility and balance:

Embrace resilience: There may be difficulties along the road, but if we are resilient and persistent, we can get beyond them and keep going in the direction of our objectives.

Celebrate progress: We should celebrate every accomplishment as we move closer to having greater flexibility and balance. Whatever our accomplishments may be, let's celebrate and recognize them.

Cultivate mindfulness: We may develop better harmony and balance in our lives and gain a deeper awareness of ourselves by being in the moment and paying attention to our bodies.

Seek support: We don't have to go through this path by ourselves. Let us turn to our family and friends for support, consult experts for advice, and establish connections with like-minded individuals.

Embrace possibilities: High potential and possibilities exist throughout the senior years. Allow us to seize the many chances for personal development and change that lie ahead as we accept new experiences and take calculated risks. Let me conclude by wishing that this book will be a source of motivation, direction, and strength for us all as we work toward living our best lives into old age with resilience, vigor, and balance.

Never forget that it is never too late to develop inner serenity, enjoy the pleasures of movement, and appreciate the beauty of life in all its forms.